SAVE MONEY

STAY

THIN

By

Dame DJ

©Dame DJ 2016

Sign up to see new releases and new Audio books

damedj@djbooks.club

To say a big 'thank you' we are sending a Free book of your choice for any Amazon kind reviews.

Just post and choose your book.

Amazon review page.

www.DJBooks.Club

Individual support & confidential discussions can be arranged.

7 days advance booking needed on GMT

Request dates via;

damedj@djbooks.club

PART 1

WHY?

WHY DO PEOPLE ON LOW INCOMES EAT CRAP?

WHY?

THEY DON'T HAVE TO.

I keep hearing the same story; that the low-income homes are more exposed to illness, likely to get fat, die early, have sick kids and end up costing the health system millions?

Why is that? I have spent the last 15 years shopping in the local markets, never buy much at the big supermarkets, have saved my self an absolute fortune and feasted on fresh wonderful produce in plentiful amounts.

What is the problem???

I just don't see it but enough people tell you there is one you will believe it in the end.

In this book I describe;

How I shop
What I pay for what
How to make decent meals for a family
Recipes
Breaking the cooking rules and thinking outside the box
Eating seasonally
How to avoid the cheap crap that is poisoning us all

If you are income-disadvantaged thing smart! Eat smart! Buy smart!

Prevent illness, prevent sickness, wake up, start peeling, start chopping and think and calculate because the way this country is going ending up in hospital could kill you!

Think before you eat.

UNDERSTANDING

We need to have an 'understanding', sing from the same hymn book and agree on some basics or this is not going to work and you don't need to read on.

We are not getting fat, compromising on health or turning to any manufactured items to save money.

We will not be buying or using any sugar.

We will be buying 'ingredients' not premade foods when possible (except things like butter pastry).

We will not use a microwave.

We will not add any tablets or powders as substitutes for food.

We will not snack in-between meals.

We will not drink any 'carbonated drinks' apart from a mineral water.

We will not buy any items that have photos OR pictures on them of the dish they hope to be.

We will not cheat or lie to our stomachs.

We will try to avoid alcohol and caffeine.

We will read food labels and try to avoid corn syrup, food additives, colorings, all E numbers, MSG and anything else that sounds chemical.

We will only use local/organic/sealed/country of origin honey and avoid all mixed/imported/blended/cheap imitations originating overseas.

We will only use fresh local garlic not garlic from China.

We will not use any cereals with added sugar/coatings or crystalized.

We will not use tinned fruits.

We will not use crisps/salted nuts/candid fruits or croutons.

We will not use any manufactured salad dressings/sauces/pickles/flavored oils or malt vinegar.

We will not use any frozen produce except peas, sweet corn, Atlantic salmon, cod, haddock or lobster.

We will not use any farmed prawns.

We will not use any pork, lamb, chicken or beef unless it's organic and has natural origins.

We will only use filtered cows milk and preferably goat's milk when possible.

We will not use any soya milks.

We will only use live unflavored natural yoghurt.

We will not use commercial cream cheeses.

We will not use/cook any margarines, or canola, palm or flavored oils.

We will not use tinned meats or fish.

We will not eat biscuits, white bread, sliced loaves, bagels etc. but only pita and sourdough bread once a week.

We will eat brown rice in preference to white when possible.

We will not drink flavored teas, cordials, squash, concentrated juices or premade smoothies, or powdered premade coffee.

We will try to drink room temperature flat mineral water when possible.

We will not use a fluoride toothpaste or cheap mouthwash.

Hunger is not a deadly pain, nothing to fear and feeling most of the world experiences daily.

I will not take it personally if you prefer to eat the above or you don't read the rest of this book.

I was forced to write this after listening to years of whining as to why income disadvantaged folks are eating crap and getting fat.

As far as I'm concerned I have *always* been income disadvantage and eat very well and am not fat. I don't understand the problem?

Lets remember the bible only had 10 commandments which considering the choices available seem now as very reasonable.

I see a lot 'stupid eating' around and wasting money and poisoning our bodies so do what you can and lets try to get as close to the goal as possible.

We need to harmonies food, eating and our relationship to this habit we encounter about 3 times a day.

Bon appetite.

BROWN RICE.

http://www.livescience.com/50461-brown-rice-health-benefits-nutrition-facts.html

Brown rice is not an option it's a must so try to include it at least once a month.

Buy and cook a bag at least once a week and have it there for all occasions especially if you have a family to feed.

Families come home hungry and don't wait around long for cooking but open fridges and cupboards look for snacks.

Brown rice is expensive but worth every penny and preferable to normal wheat gluten based pasta any day.

Info;

Brown whole grain rice, has a mild, nutty flavour, and is chewier and more nutritious than white rice unlike brown rice, has had the bran and the germ removed; and has different nutritional content.

Brown rice is a whole grain and a good source of magnesium, phosphorus, selenium, thiamine, niacin, vitamin B6, an excellent source of manganese and high in fiber.

A part of these missing nutrients, such as iron the vitamins B1 and B3 which can be added back into the white rice which the US call "enriched rice".

Magnesium is a mineral not added back into white rice.

There have been concerns over arsenic from use of inorganic arsenic as a pesticide.

Germinated grains have enzymes activated, amino acids and a nutritional advantage is brown rice that has been soaked for 4-20 hours in warm water before cooking.

The Chinese, Indian and Japanese etc. all have rice based diets with small amounts of protein and lots of vegetables but have switched from healthy brown rice to polished rice risking the health of their populations.

Having a gluten allergy is a blessing in disguise and even awareness might help us hold back from the mountains of white flour on our plates.

I don't eat rice cakes but plenty of people do.

Generally keep your starches and gluten down to a minimum but it's hard feeding a family a meal with out them as they expect them.

Info;

The story of how a once nutritious grain was transformed into something unhealthy to eat is about how corporations, and "modernization," global trade has taken over.

After farmers harvest their rice it is cleaned and the husks are taken off the grains of rice and is still is referred to as "brown rice" or "unpolished" rice. After the husk has been taken off the rice, there remain several very thin layers of wholesome bran full of nutrients, vitamins, minerals, and protein.

Years ago brown rice was called "dirty rice" but selling white form that most people prefer has caused an adverse impact on health.

We all know polishing removes most of the vitamins and minerals vital to health as the rice bran contains vitamin B and thiamine preventing beriberi.

Conditions it helps;

Harvard researchers have discovered two servings of brown rice per week can lower the risk of being diabetics but they say 50 grams of brown rice a day, lower the risk of by 16 %.

Brown rice supplies 14 % of the recommended daily value for fiber for colon cancer as the fibres tends to latch onto the chemicals that cause cancer and steer them away.

One cup of brown rice contains 88 percent of the recommended daily value of manganese, a nutrient that plays an important part in fighting free radicals. Manganese is part of a compound known as superoxide dismutase, an antioxidant that prevents damage from free radicals.

Selenium also plays a role in the antioxidant process and can destroy cancer cells and even repair DNA. Selenium is important for regulating the immune system and the thyroid hormone metabolism function.

A Harvard study shows that women who incorporate whole grains, such as brown rice, into their diet were more likely to maintain a healthy body weight.

The oil in brown rice has been shown to lower levels of LDL cholesterol, also known as the bad cholesterol, by up to seven percent.

Brown rice also have cardiovascular benefits for postmenopausal women, including slowing the build-up of plaque in the arteries, as well as slowing the progression of the narrowing of the arteries.

Phytonutrients are compounds naturally found in plants that have anti-inflammatory properties and tend to act as an antioxidant.

Metabolic syndrome is a combination of factors that increases the risk for developing type 2 diabetes, heart disease and excess fat in the abdominal area. Asthma causes many children to miss school but eating plenty of whole grains along with fish can lower the risk asthma by 30 percent.

Brown rice has magnesium essential to bone health as one cup of brown rice contains 20 percent of the recommended daily dose.

Ok, ok, ok - I got it. I *will* eat it but how?

http://www.marthastewart.com/923541/brown-rice-recipes

Put brown rice and water together in a pot with a lid. Use the ratio of 1.5 cups water to 1-cup rice.

Set the heat to maximum, and bring the rice/water to a boil uncovered.

Turn off the heat, and let the rice sit in the covered pot for another 10 minutes.

Eat and enjoy.

To Steam

Take a large pan and put olive oil, coconut oil or organic butter in the bottom.

Chop dill finely and mix into the rice

Pour the rice back onto and allow steaming on a very low heat.

Place a tea towel UNDER the lid to absorb the water so it doesn't drip back down. BE CAREFUL the towel does not set alight so fold in the entire edges well.

Its nutty steamed rice you are looking for not a burnt down house.

FISH KEGEREE

Try to get the best quality ingredients, as there aren't that many.

Naturally smoked not dyed fish & free-range eggs.

2 eggs
Spring onions
Coriander
Red chilies
Ginger

Mustards seeds
Turmeric

Fry them all gently in oil

Then add a packet of pre-cooked rice so they absorb the spices immediately

Add petit pois into the rice

Add some lemon juice

Put in the fish chunks but don't smash then up.

Chop a little coriander on top and a large knob of butter.

Pepper and salt well and serve with a side dish of a bowl of plain yogurt drizzled with sweet chili sauce

----

FISH PIE

http://www.pieminister.co.uk/food/pies/

The word 'PIE' is as over used, as the words 'love', 'diet', and 'agreement.'

Apparently the ancient Egyptians first made pies that is no surprise as if you can get a pyramid to stay up a pie is no great challenge. They used local ingredients like oats and barley and handed it down to the Greeks who thought of putting meat inside which is where we are today.

I eat very little meat and for economical purposes we are going to use frozen fish. Normally I don't like using frozen foods but the factory ships that are raping our oceans of anything left alive are packing the fish caught so fast its hardly dead and I think it's a waste to put a fresh fish hidden into a pie.

Until individual governments have the guts to changes the fishing laws and not bend to the lobbyists we have no to little chance of recovering our stocks.

I call it the 'Easter Island' argument. Some one on Easter Island said "don't cut down those remaining trees as we cant build boats and they aren't growing so fast any more" No one listened and they all ended up eating each other probably.... which bring me to another recipe.:) (Joking)

A pie can be topped with pastry, which forms a nice crust, and to me the whole point is to have the interior cooked by that crust which is also delicious to eat. It's a slow, relaxed cooking process not so sensitive and not too decorative as the more you prod the pastry on top the more rustic it looks.
Brush the top with milk at least to get the golden glow and if you prefer do a top and bottom pastry but I personally think it adds little but extra calories.

Shop bought pastry is not evil but its not the real thing for real cooks but given kitchens are small, time is short, everyone has lost the rolling pin don't feel too bad about buying the all butter roll from the supermarket.
I have in the past muddled short crust up with puff and the results have been quite tasty if not a bit different so try to use the puff for savory and the short crust for sweet pies.

Pies were for travelling and a way to transport its contents, which must have worked very well giving folks, a decent meal for days to come.

Birds were put into pies and there is a reference to a peacock pie cooked in 1429 the thought of which would fill us with horror today.

I think of pies as either 'open pies' typically filled with fruits of the season or 'closed pies' more savory using fish or meat but there are no rules just a fridge full of ingredients and hungry diners.

The 'Cornish pasty' is the hand luggage of pie making and has links to the miners whose hands were dirty so had to hold onto the crust. I don't believe it and think they were too poor to throw away a good tasty calorie filled homemade crust.

Like oriental food a pie filling can be light on the meat or fish, while heavy on vegetables then all married in a dent sauce.

Strange how you never see large pies carved up and served in decent restaurants? Occasionally one finds individual pies and of course street food has embraced the pie but what wrong with a huge great warm steaming pie for 20 in the middle of a restaurant...? Emm....

Conditions its good for;

A pumpkin pie has a following like a small religion for those who are truly converts.

- Helps cure cancer apparently
- Helps the skin
- Boosts the immune system
- High in potassium
- Great source of fiber so helps weight loss
- High in vitamin A so helps eyesight

We know that's all pumpkin related not 'pie' related but it's so popular it's worth a mention if the pumpkin is in season.

Bottom line; the pie is as healthy as what you put in it.

Ok, ok, ok I got that but how?

The easiest quickest, health pie to me is a fish pie made with frozen fish.

For about $3 a packet of mixed cod, haddock, salmon etc. cut into pieces will feed a family and it's not farmed.

Info;

Fish pie with a Thai twist.

Grease a large ovenproof dish in a large bowl mix in a selection of herbs, peppers, spices, red and greens.

Chop garlic, a couple of onions, shallots and sauté.

Use a selection of fishes salmon, cod, haddock, smoked something and mix together.

Add the onions and frozen petit pois for green.

In a small bowl pour in coconut powder and a medium spoon of Thai curry past and add a cup boiling water to mix.

Add two good spoonful's of tomatoes past to pinking the whole dish and sweeten it up.

Pour all of that over the fish and add the onions, garlic etc. and mix with a sprinkle of sea salt.

Do not add lemon or lime at this stage during the cooking it dries it out and is better squeezed on later.

Top the bowl with ($0.50 half a packet) of pastry dust over with milk so it goes golden.

Leave for 15-20 until pastry is golden brown and dust with cayenne pepper to give a red hint and more heat to the taste.

My husband used to *only* eat dishes he recognized but now he rarely eats the same dish twice and so never recognizes it which shows a great level of trust or that he's given up asking.

You can use any small fish pieces, and vary or mix up any spices.

Its fine served cold, is hard to burn, is filling, smells delicious, not fishy, not fattening, great for lunch the next day and not expensive.

Even folks who don't like fish pie like this spicy pink fish pie☺

ROAST CHICKEN

https://en.wikipedia.org/wiki/Chicken

Roast chicken is a noble and comforting dish.

Most people think making a roast lunch/diner is a big deal but really it's the easiest thing in the world and I must past on the tip my old friend gave me and gave so much joy to others.

Buy the best chicken you can afford. In France a good chicken is expensive but they value a 'poulet fermier' and I understand why.

In the UK the price of chicken has dropped over the years and they are fat, cheap and clean looking but I am afraid of what they have eaten. The yellow corn fed ones seemed to have fallen out of favor, as now we are suspicious of genetically modified corn. In the USA we used to buy Perdu chicken, which was quality, controlled and never disappointed.

Info;

In 2011 there were 19 billion chickens on earth that means somewhere there is a chicken shit mountain growing. Forget the methane the cows are belching out what and who is feeding probably 20 million birds now not many of who live beyond 3 kilos. They aren't eating the grubs and running around farms or they would occupy a landmass the entire size of Germany.

According to Columella chickens should be fed on barley groats, small chickpeas, millet and wheat bran, if they are cheap and wheat itself should be avoided, as it is harmful to the birds.

In ancient days they came from China, India, via Greece, through Egypt, Syria then up to Europe. How do we know this? We don't its just they had some ancient paintings depicting birds and we didn't.

Although they live in flocks individuals dominant in 'pecking order' and social balance is easily disturb so how they adjust to cages and isolation must be a horror.

One of the earliest records of caponisation occurred during the Roman times that disallowed fattening hens to concern rations. To get around this the Romans instead castrated roosters, which resulted in a doubling of size.

It was also practiced later throughout medieval times describing capons as preferred poultry since the ordinary fowl of the farmyard was regarded as peasant fare and "popular malice crediting monks with a weakness for capons.
You don't even want to know how this is done and is so hideous I would never eat one.

Another fine idea of man getting more after making some animals suffer.

A hen will become 'broody' and sit on clutch until they are ready and maintain their temperature and humidity but modern caged hens cannot go 'broody'.

Chickens farmed for meat are called broiler chickens. Chickens will naturally live for six or more years, but broiler chickens typically take less than six weeks to reach slaughter size. A free range or organic meat chicken will usually be slaughtered at about 14 weeks of age.

Conditions it helps are;

http://www.organicfacts.net/health-benefits/animal-product/health-benefits-of-chicken.html

Common cold; this is more to do with chicken soup but you need a chicken to make the soup so lets include it.

Weight loss; only if it's organic and not stuffed with hormones and antibiotics and all protein and white meat.

Ok, ok, ok - I got it. I *will* eat them but how?

http://www.jamieoliver.com/recipes/chicken-recipes/

Simple roast chicken

Take a large saucepan and fill with water to boil. Put in the entire chicken and bring to the boil for about 5-8 minutes.

Pour off that water.

Take a large baking tray cover with oil, species, herbs, some cut shallots, fennel, and onions

Stuff the interior of the chicken with herbs, a lemon, stuffing, peppers or something in the fridge that's fresh and natural.

Rub the skin with the oil etc. and put into the dish *upside down.*

Add a little water, cover with foil and pop into oven for 20 mins and surround the chicken with vegetables etc. to save on pans.

Remove foil, turn the chicken upright and add cheap marmalade and put back into the oven for 20 mins.

The sweet marmalade will cook quickly in the heat and bronze the skin so be careful about dropping any jus as hot sweet liquid burns.

Let it stand a minute and you will give a tasty very moist bird.

Let me know if that worked for you as my friends beg me to remake this easy dish!

ROASTED TOMATOES

http://www.whfoods.com/genpage.php?tname=foodspice&dbid=44

I love tomatoes and tomatoes love me. I should have been southern Italian and a lot of other things but lets stay on the tomatoes for now.

We grew them as kids and they climbed the wall in our small garden but I have zero recollection of ever eating them so cannot say the homegrown fruit is the best in the world. I don't think we were allowed to eat them, as they seemed a very precious and special item for a special day that never came.

Not what kids would say today I presume?

I see large bowls of cherry tomatoes and 'on the vine' tomatoes very cheap but most people just ignore them. Its like seeing Louboutins on sale, stacked on racks behind old books, and some other ordinary items...well perhaps not exactly the same but they have a red sole.

Info;

A tomatoes is a fruit and botanically and scientifically the berry-type fruits of the tomato plant, a culinary vegetable which causes confusion.

The tomato was native to western South America and was probably yellow rather than red but Europeans thought the shiny fruit was poisonous as the leaves are.

So the Aztecs grew them, then so did Mexico and then the Spanish brought them over about mid 1400. Grown in Italy by the mid 1500 they were mainly cultivated for flowers grown in beds not for food.

By the mid 1800 they were known in Britain and widely used in many dishes but mostly known from Italian and Jewish cooking.

The Brits introduced them to Aleppo in the Middle East by about 1800 where they were cultivated and used in their cuisine. Yes, the same Aleppo being bombarded today with bombs in the deathly attacks we see in Syrian on our TV.

By about 1720 they were seen in South Carolina and were still thought to be poisonous so used as an ornament plant but Thomas Jefferson ate tomatoes in Paris and sent the seeds back to the USA for cultivation.

To get the most of the sunny climates Florida and California became centres of farming and particularly concentrating on the canning process.

However now China is the world's largest producer followed by India, as it's the 8th most valuable crop in the world making the USA no 3 producer and Turkey no 4.

The largest tomatoes tree in the world may have been in Florida Disney world, which grew from seeds from China but it died in 2010.

Conditions they help;

- Studies have shown lycopene in cooked tomatoes, has been found to help prevent prostate cancer
- Very high levels of vitamin C helps the skin
- Studies show they help fight off cancer Lycopene is a natural antioxidant that works effectively to slow the growth of cancerous cells and cooked tomatoes produce even more lycopene.
- Tomatoes contain coumaric acid and chlorogenic acid that work to protect the body from carcinogens that are produced from cigarette smoke.

Vitamin B and potassium in tomatoes reduce cholesterol levels and lower blood pressure effective in prevent heart attacks, strokes as well as many other heart related problems.

- Tomatoes without seeds in some studies help reduce the risk of kidney stones.
- The Vitamin A found in tomatoes is fantastic for improving your vision. In addition, eating tomatoes is one of the best foods to eat to prevent the development of night blindness.

- Tomatoes are packed full of the valuable mineral known as chromium. It works effectively to help diabetics keep their blood sugar levels under better control.

- The Vitamin A found in tomatoes improves vision and one of the best foods to eat to prevent the development of night blindness.

- Full of the valuable mineral known as chromium they help diabetics keep their blood sugar levels under better control.

Ok, ok, ok I got it. I will eat the tomatoes but how?

http://ohsheglows.com/2012/09/05/10-tomato-recipes-to-knock-your-socks-off/

We all know about sundried tomatoes that are ridiculously expensive for a bit of 'suns shrivel' but I suppose part of that process is done by hand so the labor coast soar even if they are thrown outside over a few sheets to dry.

I have seen the women in Tunisia dry the red peppers on the floor over a couple of days that goes into the fabulous (probably cancer fighting) Harrisa which they manage to include in almost every dish.

On a tight budget these luxuries are 'walk bys' but there is an intense tasty option.

To me if you cant get the dried then roast them to intensify the flavor.

Line a big baking tray with foil to save on the scrubbing.

- Cover with oil
- Empty all the tomatoes into a bowl
- Season with plenty of interesting herbs, like;
- Herbs de Provence, sea salt, fennel seeds, couple of cloves, a bay leaf, spoonful of French mustard, spoonful of mint sauce, fresh chopped coriander, basil etc. (4 at most
- Toss together and spread into the tray with a few drops of water or vinegar (cider/ balsamic/wine only) so it doesn't dry out.
- Roast for 15 mins then toss around and another 15 mins
- Cook the pasta in hot water and add an inexpensive green/herb tea bag into the hot water (do not put pasta into cold water or add salt
- Serve over hot pasta, as a side dish, keep in the fridge, add to salads etc.
- Cost $1.50

Remember put the pasta INTO the sauce and stir in not the sauce into the pasta. That way you use the juices and don't over do the ratio with dried tasteless pasta on the bottom.

THE PERKY RADISH

I hate radishes.

I tried to like them, forced them on myself, on other people, bought them and let them shrivel in the fridge and over the years made a lot of effort to find a way to eat them.

It was like that kid at school who you were made to sit next to, tried all term to find one redeeming feature about them to enjoy only, to end up finding nothing; then understanding no one else liked them either.

I only met one man who liked radishes and I considered he had no taste, was a masochist and generally not going to live very long in life; not all those characteristics were related to his love of radishes.

But I do have good news so lets highlight *why* we should eat them seasonally.

I had noticed the markets selling two large fresh plump bunches of perky pink and confidant radishes for $1 in season. That was a good enough reason for me to try again and delve deeper into the bosom of this pink audacious root.

Info;

Radishes root vegetable belongs to the family of Brassica and enters the historical record in third century BC located the originally in Asia but the only region where truly wild forms are in central China and India, so we know they travel well! Romans in the first century gave detail small, large, round, long, mild, and sharp varieties so if the Greeks, Romans and Chinese eat them them so will I.

The radish seems to have been one of the first European crops probably because they travelled so well!

A botanist reported radishes of 100 lb. and roughly 3 ft. in length in 1544 but is that each? Like one radish? Surely not?

The only Daikon or Japanese originally cultivated on a volcanic island is the biggest in the world 6-45 kilos, which is, not surprise to me as the Japs eat horrible things.

A Chinese proverb goes like this, "eating pungent radish and drinking hot tea, let the starved doctors beg on their knees" and I bit they mean every word of it.

Radishes are a fast-growing, annual, cool-season crop and the seed germinates in three to four days and can be stored for up to two months which sounds perfect for poor communities.

Radishes can be useful as combination plants for many other crops, probably because their pungent odor deters such insect pests as aphids, and ants so function as a death trap luring insect pests away from the main crop. OK so there's the natural solution to avoiding pesticides and it's free.

Cucumbers and radishes seem to thrive when grown in close association with each other, and radishes also grow well with peas and lettuce; Its beginning to sound like a no brainer and I am already growing fond of this pink perky ball of repellant.

Names like Red King, Sicily Giant, Snow belle, Cherry Belle, French Breakfast, Plum Purple, Easter Egg and White Icicle are a lot more interesting than 'radish' and they are tasting better already!

Radish, like other cruciferous and Brassica family vegetables, contains *isothiocyanate* anti-oxidant compound. Studies suggest that sulforaphane has proven role against prostate, breast, colon and ovarian cancers by virtue of its cancer-cell growth inhibition, and cyto-toxic effects on cancer cells.

In addition, they contain adequate levels of folates, vitamin B-6, riboflavin, thiamin and minerals such as iron, magnesium, copper and calcium.

Further, they contain many phytochemicals like *indoles* that are detoxifying agents and zea-xanthin, lutein and beta-carotene, which are flavonoid antioxidants.

Conditions they help;

http://www.organicfacts.net/health-benefits/vegetable/health-benefits-of-radish.html#!

Jaundice; they help clean the liver and stomach and protects the gall bladder from infections.

Cancer; Rich in vitamin C, folic and anthocyanin's they are connected to treating colon, kidney, oral and kidney cancer as the isthiocyanates impact the genetic pathways of cancer cells causing apoptosis, call death so they don't reproduce.

Piles; Good roughage helps heal symptoms.

Urinary Disorders; they are diuretic in nature and so the juice cures inflammation and cleans out the kidneys.

Ok, ok, ok- I got it. I *will* eat them but how?

http://www.loveradish.co.uk/recipes/

Most of the recopies suggest eating them raw or steamed, which I cannot do so here's what I did discover after many trials.

Roasted Radishes.

Take an oven dish, put in oil and season well.

Top and tail washed radish and toss in the oil and oven bake for at least 30 mins.

They loose their colour and go a very pale pink.

They shrivel a bit, remind me of roasted grapes and wrinkle a bit.

Most importantly they become unrecognisable and they sweeten up and loose that bitter radish taste!

The large group of radish haters will happily scoff them down with out complaints.

Serve cut in half tossed with seeds, roasted onions or roasted red peppers.

Sprinkle with cayenne pepper or toss in Harrisa for heat and kick.

Cut up and toss into salads as they don't dominate but add fibre and crunch.

Drizzle with pomegranate molasses and serve in a bowl with toothpicks.

Delicious, so cheap and so good for you! Let us join our Chinese cousins and celebrate the radish before they take over the world☺

The other fantastic use I had for them was juicing them, which I cover in the 'Juicy You' section. Have you ever had radish juice..? No I thought not. It's delicious and doesn't taste anything like a radish!

NUTS

https://en.wikipedia.org/wiki/Nut_(fruit)

Nuts are natures super snack.

The reality is few of us know what a nut bush/tree looks like, what time of year they grow, where to find them, how to plant them, store them or even what country they come from.

It's as if they come in packets, sacs, or bins out of nowhere gathered by invisible nibble fingered people in a place we have never visited.

The walnut looks like the brain and happens to be good for the brain.

The Brazil nut tree is one of the largest in the Amazon rain forest and the nut takes 14 months to mature.

I do not agree with any salted nuts especially peanuts as the quality of the salt is low grade and the nuts could be old and harbor mould.

Info;

http://www.everydayhealth.com/diet-and-nutrition/0406/why-you-should-go-nuts-for-nuts.aspx#01

A nut in cuisine is a much less restrictive category than a nut in botany, as the term is applied to many seeds that are not botanically true nuts. Any large, oily kernels found within a shell and used in food are commonly called nuts.

Some fruits and seeds that do not meet the botanical definition but are nuts in the culinary sense is:

Almonds are the edible seeds of drupe fruits — the leathery "flesh" is removed at harvest.

Brazil nut is the seed from a capsule.

Cashew is the seed[4] of an accessory fruit.

Chilean hazelnut or Genuine

Macadamia is a creamy white kernel of a follicle type fruit.

Pecan is the seed of a drupe fruit

Peanut is a seed and from a legume type fruit (of the familyFabaceae).

Pine nut is the seed of several species.

Pistachio is the partly dehiscent seed of a thin-shelled drupe.

Walnut is the seed of a drupe fruit

Containing a relatively large quantity of calories, essential unsaturated and monounsaturated fats including linoleic acid and linolenic acid, vitamins, and essential amino acids and good source of vitamin E, vitamin B_2, folate, fiber, and the essential minerals magnesium, phosphorus, potassium, copper, and selenium.[5]

Nuts are most healthy in their raw unroasted form because up to 15% of the fats are destroyed during the roasting process

Unroasted walnuts have twice as many antioxidants as other nuts or seeds.

Conditions they help;

Eating nuts regularly can prevent coronary heart disease, ischemic heart disease, cardiovascular disease, as nuts were first linked to protection against CHD.

Consumption of almonds and walnuts can lower serum low-density lipoprotein (LDL) concentrations.

Nuts contain various substances thought to possess cardioprotective effects, their omega 3 fatty acid profile is at least in part responsible for thehypolipidemic responce and have a very low glycemic index because of their high unsaturated fat and protein content and relatively low carbohydrate content.

Nuts are included in diets for patients with insulin resistance such as Type 2 diabetes mellitus.

Nuts also help weight loss, as experts believe this is because nuts are so high in fibre; they pass through the body without being completely broken down.

Pecans are packed with plant steroid, which relieve symptoms of an enlarged prostate. Studies also found post-menopausal women with high vitamin E intake from pecans were 50 per cent less likely to die of a stroke.

A 2007 Spanish study claimed walnuts are as good as olive oil in reducing inflammation and oxidation in the arteries after a fatty meal.

Hazelnuts reduce blood cholesterol levels in men and a study found that people who ate macadamia nuts for four weeks reduced levels of blood cholesterol as they counteract the artery-blocking build-up.

Ok, ok, ok, I got it. I'm eating the nuts.

People who eat nuts tend to eat less junk food.

In Tunisia the poorest corner shops with water, soda, cigarettes and sweets still have large jars of loose nuts sold by the gram, as they are large consumers of Almonds in particular.

I was aware California had an enormous Almond production very dependent on immigrant labor I presume and highly sensitive to the long drought they are having.

Almond paste. Butter, flour, flakes, oil are a staple in a few countries and are used liberally in local foods contributing to their staple diet.

We think we have progressed so far but have replaced them with manufactured cakes, biscuits, cookies and snacks full of ingredients we cannot even pronounce and E numbers!

That's not progress!

Wash nuts and dry well before using and do not let them stay damp or go moldy unless you are soaking them over night so they germinate.

They have mostly come from 3rd world countries, were picked or shelled by hand, transported long distances in sacks potentially exposed to rats, dust and fumes.

A nut allergy is a different condition and has nothing to do with how clean a nut is. Nut allergies are on the rise and are serious and I would recommend such individuals not to go to restaurants and only eat food they have control over.

Ok, ok, ok - I got it. I *will* eat them but how?

http://www.theguardian.com/lifeandstyle/2013/apr/13/10-best-nuts-recipes

Add nuts to salads.

Add nuts to home made breads

Crush them up small in a tea towel and sprinkle over rice, pasta, potatoes etc.

Use on journeys, during the day, or at the office as emergency food.

Add mixed crushed nuts to chicken stuffing and roast.

Nuts are a constant ingredient not the main course so have them handy to add and not stuffed in the back of a pantry.

STIR FRY

SALAD

http://www.jamieoliver.com/recipes/vegetables-recipes/veggie-noodle-stir-fry/

This is one of my favourite salads and I eat it nearly every day.

Its very simple and I don't know why more people aren't eating it but I know people want the noodles more than the stir-fry. Hold the noodles until later.

When I was a child a salad was a leaf of lettuce, a couple of slices of cucumber and a slice of tomatoes *only!* And it also always had salad cream all over it. In fact it was a bowl of salad cream with some bits underneath. Terrible.

Go to the largest supermarket as they have the largest choices of pre made stir fry packets for the best price and very fresh.

Look at the oriental fresh section and find a large bag of mixed and chopped vegetables.

These will probably include;

Sliced cabbage
Carrot
Onion
Bean sprouts
Peppers

Mushroom

And anything else is a bonus.

Wash them and empty into a large bowl and make a fresh home made dressing from fresh ingredients including a spoonful of peanut butter and soy sauce.

One large bag $1.00 should feed a family of four or one large bag will provide a salad a day for 4 days; any longer and its no longer fresh enough.

Dressing $0.30

A salad is not an option and more ingredients that these are needed but it's a good base if time is short but it's not a substitute for other raw ingredients.

A salad every day at least once a day is necessary but take it a whole way further, love your salad dishes and put time into them.

It's all about going raw. A salad is a bowl of raw fruits, vegetables, leaves, nuts, seeds, sprouts, pulses, etc.

Feast in the raw and get a slicer machine if you can.

Get away from cooking/heating foods and get them fresh out of the ground and consume them fresh, alive and full of electricity.

Food is supposed to be consumed alive not dead.

Info;

Wok frying may have been used as early as the Han dynasty for drying grain not for cooking, but it was not until the Ming dynasty that the wok allowed quick cooking in hot oil.

The technique became popular because the wood and charcoal used to fire stoves were becoming increasingly expensive and stir-frying could cook food quickly without wasting fuel, which is something we need to remember too.

There are two primary techniques: *chao* and *bao* and both techniques use high heat, but *chao* adds a liquid and the ingredients are softer, where as *bao* stir fries are more crispy

Stir-frying with honey is to increase its sweetness and therefore its spleen and stomach qi tonic effects. Stir-frying in vinegar is used to direct the properties of a herb more to the liver.

So when you have left over of the salad it goes straight into the wok dressing and all.

http://www.bonappetit.com/recipes/quick-recipes/slideshow/quick-stir-fry-recipes

----

BONE BROTH SOUP

Bone broth soup is one of the funniest dishes conceived and has given me hours of amusement.

The gigantic leap man kind had to make to capture a boned animal, light a fire, bring water, develop a vessel to hold liquid and a few bits of other flavoring was probably one of his longest periods of history.

We have no idea what misery our ancestor went through to get us to the 'soup' stage and we are treating the 'bone broth' as if it's a new super food.

Did we forget they boiled leather and drank it during the siege of Leningrad?

Did we forget ancient man went months with out even catching an animal that had any bones and would have eaten insects and grubs in lean times and now we happily throw all the bones away off our plate such is the depths of our ignorance.

But I do make one exception and that is boiling the bones of farmed, caged pellet fed, hormone injected chickens. That's a chemical brew I have any intention of ingesting but we are blessed with organic produce so spend the extra and enjoy the dish.

Books on what Jewish chicken soup can cure cover every illness under the sun and we can enjoy all the folklore but beware of that chicken fat.

Many a well-meaning mother has given her husband terminal heart attacks with too much greasy fatty food.

Info;

Glycosaminoglycans (GAG) have the primary role of maintaining and supporting collagen and elastin between bones and fibers.

GAGs are supportive for digestive health restores the intestinal lining, so a deficiency is linked to digestive challenges.

Several important GAGs are found in bone broth, including glucosamine, hyaluronic acid and chondroitin sulphate.

Its endless and you need a biology degree to even being to understand what else is in bone broth and its impact on the human body;

Simply put;

If you 'believe' its good for you that thought alone will have beneficial effect.

Conditions it helps;

Heals and seals your gut as the gelatine in the bone broth found in the knuckles, feet, and other joints helps seal up holes in intestines. This helps cure chronic diarrhoea, constipation, and even some food intolerances.

Protect your joints. Taking glucosamine supplements to help with joint pain has been common knowledge for years, but it turns out that bone broth has glucosamine too. The chondroitin sulfate in bone broth has been shown to help prevent osteoarthritis.

Bone broth is a rich source of collagen. You can find collagen in all kinds of "plumping" products these days, but why stick it on the outside when you can drink it?

Sleeping better as the glycine in bone broth has been shown in several studies to help people sleep better and improve memory.

Immune support refers to bone broth a "superfood" thanks to the high concentration of minerals and bone marrow can help strengthen your immune system.

Stronger bones as the phosphorus, magnesium, and calcium in the bones seeps out into the broth provide the body with nutrients essential for healthy bones.

Ok, ok ok. I got that but how?

http://nourishedkitchen.com/bone-broth/

In a large pan, gently fry the onions, garlic, leeks, or shallots in ghee or olive oil until soft – but not brown – about 6 minutes.

Add the meat of choice preferable grass fed neck of lamb, organic meat or chicken and fry for another 5 mins to bronze.

Add carrots, broccoli, cabbage & celery, stir and let them fry for 4 minutes. Then add finely chopped coriander stems, fines herb, turmeric, harrisa, salt, pepper, and cumin and fennel seeds.

Pour in 1-2 pints of water depending on the pan.

Stir in a good amount of tomatoes paste, a dash of pomegranate molasses or fig balsamic (something sweet) plus a good stick of cinnamon.

Bring to the boil and leave for 10 mins.

Turn it down to simmer for at least 30 mins.

Leave to stand most of the day and re heat when ready to serve.

A good soup takes time to marry.

If you enjoy what you are eating it will be a sensual worthwhile preparation and a pleasure worth sharing.

Cook other foods **in** the bone broth; pasta, rice, fish, vegetables, noddle's and anything else you would normally boil in water.

Boil the bones then cool and store in a large jar in the fridge and add to many other dishes before even starting on a soup itself.

Very few bone broths taste the same so relish and enjoy the best formula you can make.

SOUP

Goes into the

COUSCOUS.

We all know how a soup just gets better, more intense and full of subtle flavors as time goes on.

Save the last 2-4 inches of soup in the saucepan and heat up with or with the bits of vegetables (no bones).

At about boiling point tip in half a packet of couscous and stir.

Add a little olive oil for lubrication and let the couscous absorb the juices.

Turn off and serve hot or cold.

It's almost impossible to get such intensity if you start the other way around with couscous into plain water *then* add the spices.

Rationally in Tunisia they rub the dry couscous with lots olive oil then put it into a steamer placed *over* lamb cooking in harrisa and spices so it absorbs the steam and remains fluffy.

Spritz some lemon juice and a small blob of harrisa over for extra fizz. Top with plain yogurt if desired.

Couscous half a packet $0.60.

The soup was free.

ROASTED FRUIT

http://www.wholefoodsmarket.com/blog/kitchen-basics-roasting-fall-fruits

Why aren't we roasting more fruit?

Roast what's in season, cheap and plentiful obviously not the expensive out of season precious rare fruits.

That's obvious but what wrong with eating with the seasons?

We are supposed to be doing exactly that, as we are not divorced from the harvest around us!

Is it because fruit is so expensive we want to eat it fresh?

Is it because drying it is the natural preservative in times of plenty? And if that so why is dried fruit so expensive? And we seem to use that in such small amounts?

Ever since we joined the EU no country seems to have an abundant harvest and no far off country seems too able to offload any cheap plentiful harvests. Never!

Its only in the open air markets one can get a deal on either a seasonal fruit, unripen fruit or over ripe fruit.

If you buy some fruits under ripe they *cannot and won't* ripen even in the sun so try avoiding them.

Put any hard un ripened food outside in the sun for a day or by a window to get max light exposure.

Conditions they help;

http://www.theimpeccableplate.com/blog/2015/03/20/raw-versus-cooked-fruits-and-vegetables/

Pigments called anthocyanins give red and purple fruits and vegetables their color and serve as powerful antioxidants and maintain a healthy heart and improving memory function.

Studies show anthocyanins decrease the risk of macular degeneration, certain types of cancer.

Strawberries are good sources of folic acid.

Cranberries, strawberries, raspberries, red or pink grapefruit, blueberries, peppers all are loaded with vitamin C.

Cherries, prunes, peaches have plenty of fiber.

Cranberries contain a compound that prevents bacteria from sticking to the bladder walls, protect against urinary tract infections.

Certain other red or purple fruits and vegetables are particularly important for people who have diabetes.

Cherries, figs, and tomatoes are high in potassium—a mineral that helps lower blood pressure.

Nutrients found in orange and yellow fruits and veggies include vitamin C, potassium, folic acid, and bromelaine. Oranges might be the most common fruit we eat for vitamin C, but it's also present cantaloupe, peaches, mangoes, and papaya.

I rest my case -we don't need to hear much more.

Items I found 20th May 2016 for $1.45 (£1) each;

I pineapple (£0.69)
A big bowl of grapes (2 lbs)
7 pears
6 Pink Lady apples
6 Golden delicious apples
8 bananas
2 punets of strawberries
8 bananas
8 kiwis
6 plums
6 lemons

4 large oranges

Large bowl of cherry tomatoes (which are fruits)

8 tangerines

5 limes

3 grapefruit

Bowl of blueberries

Take a large oven dish and a large knob of coconut oil.

Sprinkle in cinnamon, a few cloves and pinch of salt.

Chop and spread the fruits –including the grapes- all over and add a drop of water.

Into the oven for 10 mins and turn over for another 10 mins and let the flavors intensify.

*Or make skewers of copped lumps of pineapple, apples, bananas, dates, pears etc.

*Or stew left over fruits in a saucepan with a little water on a gentle heat until soft and store in the fridge. Perfect for breakfast with yoghurt.

Sweeten with natural organic local honey, rose water, geranium water, date or pomegranate molasses, and decimated coconut *if* needed.

Add to meat dishes, chicken dishes, chop into brown rice, blend into smoothies, top with yogurt, add to cereal, leave out cold for snacks, chop into salads, perfect for older folks with no teeth.

Do not add sugar please-we don't buy or have any sugar in the house...right?

Extensive diet, nutrition and wellness research on Wikipedia and Google.

To say a big 'thank you' we are sending a Free book of your choice for any Amazon kind reviews.

Just post and choose a book.

Amazon review page.

About the Author

Dame DJ

Please join us at

www. DJBooks.Club

Sign up for a free eBook

Contact;

damedj@DJBooks.club

Dame DJ describes herself as "married young, divorced young, had two children young, starved young, remarried a couple more times, & lived in different countries to learn about life"

'Downsize to Freedom' FREE Part 1 (Part 2 out now) eBook was written after liquidating, removing all financial obligations, selling overpriced assets and "downsizing" - to everyone's horror.

https://amzn.com/B011UT6RNS

AUDIO BOOK to be released in June 2016

Gourmands on the Run! FREE Part 1 (Part 2 out now) Is a diary of an English woman on a car journey through France, from Paris to Monaco visiting the best hotels & restaurants and illustrated with her original watercolors.

https://amzn.com/B0158ZJU7A

AUDIO BOOK by Sharon Hoyland.

'To be, or not to be Single. That is my Question?' FREE Part 1 (Part 2 out now) eBook is about going in, and coming out of relationships, with some damage control.

https://amzn.com/B01577WPZ8

AUDIO BOOK by John Bico

'Percy the Pea and Other Friends' FREE eBook is a children's eBook about healthy eating and illustrated with her own watercolor paintings.

https://amzn.com/B015D5W0E0

AUDIO BOOK for kids by Dorothy Deavers.

'Behind the Wall' FREE PART 1 (Part 2 & 3 out now) is a factual eBook story describing an English woman's t revelations about moving into a luxury Florida gated golf community.

AUDIO BOOK by Frankie Wyck

The Dope Diet' new FREE Part 1 (Part 2 out now) Ebook
The 'The Dope Diet' is an intimate diary of a young English man David
Grey and his struggles with smoking dope.
Tragically he lost more than 8 kilos, money, family, friends and nearly
his sanity during his journey, crusade for legalization and acceptance.

Our guest author is

DAVID GREY

New book

THE POT HOLE

A Pot Delusion.

David Grey gives us a very personal and revealing account of his two-year drug habit in The Pot Hole as he describes his marijuana use, its potential addictiveness and consequences many pot smokers are likely to suffer. David's honest insight into his conflict of wanting to advocate the legality and end prohibition of marijuana whilst struggling with the personal conflicts brought on by the dependence on a destructive drug habit. The Pot Hole gives us a fascinating intimate glimpse into the mind of a pot user and illustrates the conflicting perspectives of addiction and the powerful seduction of this forbidden plant. Following him for two years from his initial introduction by his pretty girlfriend CC in romantic Barcelona to isolation in a French mountain village we journey with him along a bumpy route all too familiar with drug issues.

Individual support & confidential discussions can be
arranged details on

www.DJBooks.Club

7 days advance booking needed on GMT

per hour non-members

half price 1stday of every month

Request dates via;

damedj@DJBooks.Club

Join us on Twitter

@PercyThePea

@GourmandsOnRun

@NotToBeSingle

@DownsizeToFree

@_Behind_TheWall

@thedopediet

@davidgrey999